Dear Reader,

This book has been created with love and dedicati....ave created this health history book based upon what I want in it for my family.

When we visit the doctors' office, doctors often have limited amounts of time to help us. Therefore, we need to address our concerns within a short amount of time. This book will provide the information you need to partner with your doctor in achieving an accurate diagnosis.

I have created a book with fast information at your finger tips. You can take charge of your own health and the health of your loved ones. When a loved one becomes ill, we often want to help them get well. So often we forget the symptoms they had or ailments they experienced. This book will help keep track of symptoms to help ensure a proper diagnosis. For family members with severe illness, you will be able to keep track of all the doctor appointments, medications and ailments all in one place. I have created this book with places to write page numbers for cross referencing and I have made it easy to use for quick access to the information.

This book will help you record the health history for each member of your family. What a blessing this will be to a child someday. Instead of attempting to pass down health history information years after its occurrence and assuming you will be around when your child needs to know the information, you can now hand your son or daughter their own health history book. No longer will they have to rely on your physical presence to help them answer questions like, "Did I have the same illness my child has when I was young?".

It is good to track your medical history regardless of whether a family member (or yourself) is healthy or ill. This book will provide the information you need quickly without spending inordinate amounts of time looking information up.

I have created a book to benefit you and your family richly. Consider purchasing one for each member of your family and for gifts (such as baby shower, wedding, or birthdays).

Many blessings & I wish your family future health.

Sincerely,

Sarah Holmes

_____'s Health History

From:_____ To:_____

List of Current Doctors

Doctor	Specialty	Phone Number	Address	Date Acquired	Current?

Important Information for Caretakers

Birthdate_____

Address_____

_____

_____

_____

_____

Phone Number_____

Insurance_____

_____

Next of Kin Name_____

Relationship_____ Phone Number_____

Address_____

_____

_____

_____

_____

Other_____

_____

_____

Table of Contents

Records of Dr. Appointments

Date	Doctor	Reason for Appt.	Medication	Related Pages

Records of Dr. Appointments

Date	Doctor	Reason for Appt.	Medication	Related Pages

Records of Dr. Appointments

Date	Doctor	Reason for Appt.	Medication	Related Pages

Records of Ailments

Date	Description of Ailment	Treatment/ Medication	Cause	Related Pages
-------	Ex: Left Wrist Pain - Tingling	Ex: Stopped Typing & Took IbuProfen	Ex: Typed for 2 Hrs Prior to Pain	-------

Records of Ailments

Date	Description of Ailment	Treatment/ Medication	Cause	Related Pages
-------	Ex: Left Wrist Pain - Tingling	Ex: Stopped Typing & Took 2 IbuProfen	Ex: Typed for 2 Hrs Prior to Pain	

Records of Ailments

Date	Description of Ailment	Treatment/ Medication	Cause	Related Pages
-------	Ex: Left Wrist Pain - Tingling	Ex: Stopped Typing & Took 2 IbuProfen	Ex: Typed for 2 Hrs Prior to Pain	

Records of Ailments

Date	Description of Ailment	Treatment/ Medication	Cause	Related Pages
-------	Ex: Left Wrist Pain - Tingling	Ex: Stopped Typing & Took 2 IbuProfen	Ex: Typed for 2 Hrs Prior to Pain	

Records of Ailments

Date	Description of Ailment	Treatment/ Medication	Cause	Related Pages
-------	Ex: Left Wrist Pain - Tingling	Ex: Stopped Typing & Took 2 IbuProfen	Ex: Typed for 2 Hrs Prior to Pain	

Records of Ailments

Date	Description of Ailment	Treatment/ Medication	Cause	Related Pages
-------	Ex: Left Wrist Pain - Tingling	Ex: Stopped Typing & Took 2 IbuProfen	Ex: Typed for 2 Hrs Prior to Pain	

Records of Ailments

Date	Description of Ailment	Treatment/ Medication	Cause	Related Pages
-------	Ex: Left Wrist Pain - Tingling	Ex: Stopped Typing & Took 2 IbuProfen	Ex: Typed for 2 Hrs Prior to Pain	

Records of Ailments

Date	Description of Ailment	Treatment/ Medication	Cause	Related Pages
-------	Ex: Left Wrist Pain - Tingling	Ex: Stopped Typing & Took 2 IbuProfen	Ex: Typed for 2 Hrs Prior to Pain	

Records of Ailments

Date	Description of Ailment	Treatment/ Medication	Cause	Related Pages
-------	Ex: Left Wrist Pain - Tingling	Ex: Stopped Typing & Took 2 IbuProfen	Ex: Typed for 2 Hrs Prior to Pain	

Records of Ailments

Date	Description of Ailment	Treatment/ Medication	Cause	Related Pages
-------	Ex: Left Wrist Pain - Tingling	Ex: Stopped Typing & Took 2 IbuProfen	Ex: Typed for 2 Hrs Prior to Pain	

Records of Dr. Appointments

Date	Doctor	Reason for Appt.	Medication	Related Pages

Records of Dr. Appointments

Date	Doctor	Reason for Appt.	Medication	Related Pages

Records of Dr. Appointments

Date	Doctor	Reason for Appt.	Medication	Related Pages

Records of Dr. Appointments

Date	Doctor	Reason for Appt.	Medication	Related Pages

Records of Dr. Appointments

Date	Doctor	Reason for Appt.	Medication	Related Pages

Records of Dr. Appointments

Date	Doctor	Reason for Appt.	Medication	Related Pages

Records of Dr. Appointments

Date	Doctor	Reason for Appt.	Medication	Related Pages

Records of Dr. Appointments

Date	Doctor	Reason for Appt.	Medication	Related Pages

Records of Dr. Appointments

Date	Doctor	Reason for Appt.	Medication	Related Pages

Records of Dr. Appointments

Date	Doctor	Reason for Appt.	Medication	Related Pages

Records of Dr. Appointments

Date	Doctor	Reason for Appt.	Medication	Related Pages

Vaccination History

Date	Vaccination	Type of Vaccination	Doctor	Referring Pages
----------	Ex: Mumps	Ex: Oral or Shot	Ex: Dr. Smith	Ex: Pg. 10 Appt

List of Current Medication

Date	Ailment	Medication	Dosage	Doctor	Precautions/ Extra Info	Related Page Numbers

List of Current Medication

Date Acquired	Medication	Dosage	Reason for Taking	Possible Side Effects	Current?

List of Current Medication

Date Acquired	Medication	Dosage	Reason for Taking	Possible Side Effects	Current?

List of Current Medication

Date Acquired	Medication	Dosage	Reason for Taking	Possible Side Effects	Current?

List of Current Medication

Date Acquired	Medication	Dosage	Reason for Taking	Possible Side Effects	Current?

Date_____   Event:_____

Health Notes:_____

_____

_____

_____

_____

_____

_____

_____

_____

_____

_____

_____

_____

_____

_____

_____

_____

_____

_____

_____

_____

_____

_____

_____

_____

_____

_____

_____

_____

_____

_____

_____

Related Pages:_____

Date_____   Event:_____

Health Notes:_____

_____

_____

_____

_____

_____

_____

_____

_____

_____

_____

_____

_____

_____

_____

_____

_____

_____

_____

_____

_____

_____

_____

_____

_____

Related Pages:_____

Date_____   Event:_____

Health Notes:_____

_____
_____
_____
_____
_____
_____
_____
_____
_____
_____
_____
_____
_____
_____
_____
_____
_____
_____
_____
_____
_____
_____
_____
_____
_____
_____
_____
_____
_____

Related Pages:_____

Date_____   Event:_____

Health Notes:_____

_____

_____

_____

_____

_____

_____

_____

_____

_____

_____

_____

_____

_____

_____

_____

_____

_____

_____

_____

_____

_____

_____

_____

_____

_____

_____

_____

Related Pages:_____

Date_____   Event:_____

Health Notes:_____

_____

_____

_____

_____

_____

_____

_____

_____

_____

_____

_____

_____

_____

_____

_____

_____

_____

_____

_____

_____

_____

_____

_____

_____

_____

_____

_____

_____

_____

_____

Related Pages:_____

Date_____   Event:_____

Health Notes:_____

_____

_____

_____

_____

_____

_____

_____

_____

_____

_____

_____

_____

_____

_____

_____

_____

_____

_____

_____

_____

_____

_____

_____

_____

_____

_____

_____

_____

Related Pages:_____

Date_____   Event:_____

Health Notes:_____

_____

_____

_____

_____

_____

_____

_____

_____

_____

_____

_____

_____

_____

_____

_____

_____

_____

_____

_____

_____

_____

_____

_____

_____

_____

_____

_____

_____

Related Pages:_____

Date_____ Event:_____

Health Notes:_____

_____

_____

_____

_____

_____

_____

_____

_____

_____

_____

_____

_____

_____

_____

_____

_____

_____

_____

_____

_____

_____

_____

_____

_____

_____

_____

Related Pages:_____

Date_____   Event:_____

Health Notes:_____

_____

_____

_____

_____

_____

_____

_____

_____

_____

_____

_____

_____

_____

_____

_____

_____

_____

_____

_____

_____

_____

_____

_____

_____

_____

_____

_____

_____

_____

Related Pages:_____

Date_____ Event:_____

Health Notes:_____

_____
_____
_____
_____
_____
_____
_____
_____
_____
_____
_____
_____
_____
_____
_____
_____
_____
_____
_____
_____
_____
_____
_____
_____
_____
_____
_____
_____

Related Pages:_____

Date_____   Event:_____

Health Notes:_____

_____

_____

_____

_____

_____

_____

_____

_____

_____

_____

_____

_____

_____

_____

_____

_____

_____

_____

_____

_____

_____

_____

_____

_____

_____

_____

_____

_____

Related Pages:_____

Date_____   Event:_____

Health Notes:_____
_____
_____
_____
_____
_____
_____
_____
_____
_____
_____
_____
_____
_____
_____
_____
_____
_____
_____
_____
_____
_____
_____
_____
_____
_____
_____
_____
_____
_____
_____

Related Pages:_____

Date_____   Event:_____

Health Notes:_____

_____

_____

_____

_____

_____

_____

_____

_____

_____

_____

_____

_____

_____

_____

_____

_____

_____

_____

_____

_____

_____

_____

_____

_____

_____

_____

_____

_____

Related Pages:_____

Date_____   Event:_____

Health Notes:_____

_____
_____
_____
_____
_____
_____
_____
_____
_____
_____
_____
_____
_____
_____
_____
_____
_____
_____
_____
_____
_____
_____
_____
_____
_____
_____
_____
_____

Related Pages:_____

Date_____   Event:_____

Health Notes:_____

_____

_____

_____

_____

_____

_____

_____

_____

_____

_____

_____

_____

_____

_____

_____

_____

_____

_____

_____

_____

_____

_____

_____

_____

_____

_____

Related Pages:_____

Date_____   Event:_____

Health Notes:_____

_____

_____

_____

_____

_____

_____

_____

_____

_____

_____

_____

_____

_____

_____

_____

_____

_____

_____

_____

_____

_____

_____

_____

_____

_____

_____

Related Pages:_____

Date_____   Event:_____

Health Notes:_____

_____

_____

_____

_____

_____

_____

_____

_____

_____

_____

_____

_____

_____

_____

_____

_____

_____

_____

_____

_____

_____

_____

_____

_____

Related Pages:_____

Date_____   Event:_____

Health Notes:_____

_____
_____
_____
_____
_____
_____
_____
_____
_____
_____
_____
_____
_____
_____
_____
_____
_____
_____
_____
_____
_____
_____
_____
_____
_____
_____
_____
_____
_____
_____
_____

Related Pages:_____

Date_____   Event:_____

Health Notes:_____

_____

_____

_____

_____

_____

_____

_____

_____

_____

_____

_____

_____

_____

_____

_____

_____

_____

_____

_____

_____

_____

_____

_____

_____

_____

_____

_____

Related Pages:_____

Date_____   Event:_____

Health Notes:_____

_____

_____

_____

_____

_____

_____

_____

_____

_____

_____

_____

_____

_____

_____

_____

_____

_____

_____

_____

_____

_____

_____

_____

_____

_____

_____

_____

_____

Related Pages:_____

Date_____   Event:_____

Health Notes:_____

_____
_____
_____
_____
_____
_____
_____
_____
_____
_____
_____
_____
_____
_____
_____
_____
_____
_____
_____
_____
_____
_____
_____
_____
_____
_____
_____
_____
_____
_____

Related Pages:_____

Date_____   Event:_____

Health Notes:_____

_____

_____

_____

_____

_____

_____

_____

_____

_____

_____

_____

_____

_____

_____

_____

_____

_____

_____

_____

_____

_____

_____

_____

_____

_____

_____

_____

_____

Related Pages:_____

Date_____   Event:_____

Health Notes:_____

_____

_____

_____

_____

_____

_____

_____

_____

_____

_____

_____

_____

_____

_____

_____

_____

_____

_____

_____

_____

_____

_____

_____

_____

_____

_____

_____

_____

_____

_____

_____

Related Pages:_____

Date_____   Event:_____

Health Notes:_____

_____
_____
_____
_____
_____
_____
_____
_____
_____
_____
_____
_____
_____
_____
_____
_____
_____
_____
_____
_____
_____
_____
_____
_____
_____
_____
_____
_____
_____

Related Pages:_____

Date_____   Event:_____

Health Notes:_____

_____

_____

_____

_____

_____

_____

_____

_____

_____

_____

_____

_____

_____

_____

_____

_____

_____

_____

_____

_____

_____

_____

_____

_____

_____

_____

_____

_____

_____

_____

Related Pages:_____

Date_____   Event:_____

Health Notes:_____

_____

_____

_____

_____

_____

_____

_____

_____

_____

_____

_____

_____

_____

_____

_____

_____

_____

_____

_____

_____

_____

_____

_____

_____

_____

_____

Related Pages:_____

Date_____ Event:_____

Health Notes:_____

_____
_____
_____
_____
_____
_____
_____
_____
_____
_____
_____
_____
_____
_____
_____
_____
_____
_____
_____
_____
_____
_____
_____
_____
_____
_____
_____
_____
_____
_____
_____

Related Pages:_____

Date_____   Event:_____

Health Notes:_____

_____
_____
_____
_____
_____
_____
_____
_____
_____
_____
_____
_____
_____
_____
_____
_____
_____
_____
_____
_____
_____
_____
_____
_____
_____
_____
_____
_____
_____

Related Pages:_____

Date_____   Event:_____

Health Notes:_____

_____

_____

_____

_____

_____

_____

_____

_____

_____

_____

_____

_____

_____

_____

_____

_____

_____

_____

_____

_____

_____

_____

_____

_____

_____

_____

_____

Related Pages:_____

Date_____   Event:_____

Health Notes:_____

_____

_____

_____

_____

_____

_____

_____

_____

_____

_____

_____

_____

_____

_____

_____

_____

_____

_____

_____

_____

_____

_____

_____

_____

_____

_____

_____

_____

Related Pages:_____

Date_____   Event:_____

Health Notes:_____

_____

_____

_____

_____

_____

_____

_____

_____

_____

_____

_____

_____

_____

_____

_____

_____

_____

_____

_____

_____

_____

_____

_____

_____

_____

_____

_____

_____

_____

_____

Related Pages:_____

Date_____   Event:_____

Health Notes:_____

_____

_____

_____

_____

_____

_____

_____

_____

_____

_____

_____

_____

_____

_____

_____

_____

_____

_____

_____

_____

_____

_____

_____

_____

_____

_____

_____

_____

Related Pages:_____

Date_____   Event:_____

Health Notes:_____

_____
_____
_____
_____
_____
_____
_____
_____
_____
_____
_____
_____
_____
_____
_____
_____
_____
_____
_____
_____
_____
_____
_____
_____
_____
_____
_____
_____
_____

Related Pages:_____

Date_____   Event:_____

Health Notes:_____

_____
_____
_____
_____
_____
_____
_____
_____
_____
_____
_____
_____
_____
_____
_____
_____
_____
_____
_____
_____
_____
_____
_____
_____
_____
_____
_____
_____
_____
_____
_____

Related Pages:_____

Date_____   Event:_____

Health Notes:_____

_____

_____

_____

_____

_____

_____

_____

_____

_____

_____

_____

_____

_____

_____

_____

_____

_____

_____

_____

_____

_____

_____

_____

_____

_____

_____

_____

_____

Related Pages:_____

Date_____   Event:_____

Health Notes:_____

_____
_____
_____
_____
_____
_____
_____
_____
_____
_____
_____
_____
_____
_____
_____
_____
_____
_____
_____
_____
_____
_____
_____
_____
_____
_____
_____
_____
_____

Related Pages:_____

Date_____   Event:_____

Health Notes:_____

_____

_____

_____

_____

_____

_____

_____

_____

_____

_____

_____

_____

_____

_____

_____

_____

_____

_____

_____

_____

_____

_____

_____

_____

_____

_____

_____

_____

_____

_____

Related Pages:_____

Date_____   Event:_____

Health Notes:_____

_____

_____

_____

_____

_____

_____

_____

_____

_____

_____

_____

_____

_____

_____

_____

_____

_____

_____

_____

_____

_____

_____

_____

_____

_____

_____

_____

Related Pages:_____

Date_____   Event:_____

Health Notes:_____

_____
_____
_____
_____
_____
_____
_____
_____
_____
_____
_____
_____
_____
_____
_____
_____
_____
_____
_____
_____
_____
_____
_____
_____
_____
_____
_____
_____
_____
_____
_____

Related Pages:_____

Date_____   Event:_____

Health Notes:_____

_____

_____

_____

_____

_____

_____

_____

_____

_____

_____

_____

_____

_____

_____

_____

_____

_____

_____

_____

_____

_____

_____

_____

_____

_____

_____

_____

_____

_____

Related Pages:_____

Date_____   Event:_____

Health Notes:_____

_____

_____

_____

_____

_____

_____

_____

_____

_____

_____

_____

_____

_____

_____

_____

_____

_____

_____

_____

_____

_____

_____

_____

_____

_____

_____

_____

_____

_____

_____

_____

Related Pages:_____

Date_____   Event:_____

Health Notes:_____

_____

_____

_____

_____

_____

_____

_____

_____

_____

_____

_____

_____

_____

_____

_____

_____

_____

_____

_____

_____

_____

_____

_____

_____

_____

_____

_____

Related Pages:_____

Date_____   Event:_____

Health Notes:_____

_____

_____

_____

_____

_____

_____

_____

_____

_____

_____

_____

_____

_____

_____

_____

_____

_____

_____

_____

_____

_____

_____

_____

_____

_____

_____

_____

_____

_____

_____

_____

Related Pages:_____

Date_____   Event:_____

Health Notes:_____

_____
_____
_____
_____
_____
_____
_____
_____
_____
_____
_____
_____
_____
_____
_____
_____
_____
_____
_____
_____
_____
_____
_____
_____
_____
_____
_____

Related Pages:_____

Date_____   Event:_____

Health Notes:_____

_____
_____
_____
_____
_____
_____
_____
_____
_____
_____
_____
_____
_____
_____
_____
_____
_____
_____
_____
_____
_____
_____
_____
_____
_____
_____
_____
_____
_____
_____
_____
_____

Related Pages:_____

Date_____   Event:_____

Health Notes:_____

_____

_____

_____

_____

_____

_____

_____

_____

_____

_____

_____

_____

_____

_____

_____

_____

_____

_____

_____

_____

_____

_____

_____

_____

_____

_____

_____

_____

_____

_____

Related Pages:_____

Date_____   Event:_____

Health Notes:_____

_____

_____

_____

_____

_____

_____

_____

_____

_____

_____

_____

_____

_____

_____

_____

_____

_____

_____

_____

_____

_____

_____

_____

_____

_____

_____

_____

_____

_____

_____

_____

Related Pages:_____

Date_____ Event:_____

Health Notes:_____

_____

_____

_____

_____

_____

_____

_____

_____

_____

_____

_____

_____

_____

_____

_____

_____

_____

_____

_____

_____

_____

_____

_____

_____

_____

_____

_____

_____

_____

_____

Related Pages:_____

Date_____   Event:_____

Health Notes:_____

_____

_____

_____

_____

_____

_____

_____

_____

_____

_____

_____

_____

_____

_____

_____

_____

_____

_____

_____

_____

_____

_____

_____

_____

_____

_____

_____

_____

_____

_____

_____

Related Pages:_____

Date_____   Event:_____

Health Notes:_____

_____

_____

_____

_____

_____

_____

_____

_____

_____

_____

_____

_____

_____

_____

_____

_____

_____

_____

_____

_____

_____

_____

_____

_____

_____

_____

_____

_____

Related Pages:_____

Date_____   Dr:_____ Dr. Ph. No._____

Illness/Problem:_____

_____

_____

_____

Diagnosis:_____

_____

_____

_____

_____

_____

_____

_____

_____

_____

Treatment:_____

_____

_____

_____

_____

_____

_____

_____

_____

_____

_____

Medication/Dosage:_____

_____

_____

_____

_____

_____

Date_____   Dr:_____ Dr. Ph. No._____

Illness/Problem:_____
_____
_____
_____

Diagnosis:_____
_____
_____
_____
_____
_____
_____
_____
_____
_____

Treatment:_____
_____
_____
_____
_____
_____
_____
_____
_____
_____
_____
_____

Medication/Dosage:_____
_____
_____
_____
_____
_____

Date_____   Dr:_____ Dr. Ph. No._____

Illness/Problem:_____

_____

_____

_____

Diagnosis:_____

_____

_____

_____

_____

_____

_____

_____

_____

_____

Treatment:_____

_____

_____

_____

_____

_____

_____

_____

_____

_____

_____

_____

Medication/Dosage:_____

_____

_____

_____

_____

_____

Date_____   Dr:_____ Dr. Ph. No._____

Illness/Problem:_____

_____

_____

_____

Diagnosis:_____

_____

_____

_____

_____

_____

_____

_____

_____

Treatment:_____

_____

_____

_____

_____

_____

_____

_____

_____

_____

_____

Medication/Dosage:_____

_____

_____

_____

_____

_____

Date_____   Dr:_____ Dr. Ph. No._____

Illness/Problem:_____

_____

_____

_____

Diagnosis:_____

_____

_____

_____

_____

_____

_____

_____

_____

_____

Treatment:_____

_____

_____

_____

_____

_____

_____

_____

_____

_____

_____

Medication/Dosage:_____

_____

_____

_____

_____

_____

Date_____   Dr:_____ Dr. Ph. No._____

Illness/Problem:_____

_____

_____

_____

Diagnosis:_____

_____

_____

_____

_____

_____

_____

_____

_____

_____

Treatment:_____

_____

_____

_____

_____

_____

_____

_____

_____

_____

_____

_____

Medication/Dosage:_____

_____

_____

_____

_____

_____

Date_____   Dr:_____ Dr. Ph. No._____

Illness/Problem:_____

_____

_____

_____

Diagnosis:_____

_____

_____

_____

_____

_____

_____

_____

_____

_____

Treatment:_____

_____

_____

_____

_____

_____

_____

_____

_____

_____

_____

_____

_____

Medication/Dosage:_____

_____

_____

_____

_____

_____

_____

Date_____   Dr:_____ Dr. Ph. No._____

Illness/Problem:_____

_____

_____

_____

Diagnosis:_____

_____

_____

_____

_____

_____

_____

_____

_____

_____

Treatment:_____

_____

_____

_____

_____

_____

_____

_____

_____

_____

_____

_____

Medication/Dosage:_____

_____

_____

_____

_____

_____

Date_____   Dr:_____ Dr. Ph. No._____

Illness/Problem:_____

_____

_____

_____

Diagnosis:_____

_____

_____

_____

_____

_____

_____

_____

_____

_____

Treatment:_____

_____

_____

_____

_____

_____

_____

_____

_____

_____

_____

Medication/Dosage:_____

_____

_____

_____

_____

_____

Date_____   Dr:_____ Dr. Ph. No._____

Illness/Problem:_____
_____
_____
_____

Diagnosis:_____
_____
_____
_____
_____
_____
_____
_____
_____
_____
_____

Treatment:_____
_____
_____
_____
_____
_____
_____
_____
_____
_____
_____
_____
_____
_____

Medication/Dosage:_____
_____
_____
_____
_____
_____
_____

Date_____   Dr:_____ Dr. Ph. No._____

Illness/Problem:_____

_____

_____

_____

Diagnosis:_____

_____

_____

_____

_____

_____

_____

_____

_____

Treatment:_____

_____

_____

_____

_____

_____

_____

_____

_____

_____

_____

Medication/Dosage:_____

_____

_____

_____

_____

_____

Date_____   Dr:_____ Dr. Ph. No._____

Illness/Problem:_____
_____
_____
_____

Diagnosis:_____
_____
_____
_____
_____
_____
_____
_____
_____
_____

Treatment:_____
_____
_____
_____
_____
_____
_____
_____
_____
_____
_____
_____
_____

Medication/Dosage:_____
_____
_____
_____
_____
_____

Date_____   Dr:_____ Dr. Ph. No._____

Illness/Problem:_____

_____

_____

_____

Diagnosis:_____

_____

_____

_____

_____

_____

_____

_____

_____

_____

Treatment:_____

_____

_____

_____

_____

_____

_____

_____

_____

_____

Medication/Dosage:_____

_____

_____

_____

_____

_____

Date_____   Dr:_____ Dr. Ph. No._____

Illness/Problem:_____

_____

_____

_____

Diagnosis:_____

_____

_____

_____

_____

_____

_____

_____

_____

_____

Treatment:_____

_____

_____

_____

_____

_____

_____

_____

_____

_____

_____

_____

_____

_____

Medication/Dosage:_____

_____

_____

_____

_____

_____

Date_____ Dr:_____ Dr. Ph. No._____

Illness/Problem:_____
_____
_____
_____

Diagnosis:_____
_____
_____
_____
_____
_____
_____
_____
_____
_____

Treatment:_____
_____
_____
_____
_____
_____
_____
_____
_____
_____
_____
_____

Medication/Dosage:_____
_____
_____
_____
_____
_____

Date_____ Dr:_____ Dr. Ph. No._____

Illness/Problem:_____

_____

_____

_____

Diagnosis:_____

_____

_____

_____

_____

_____

_____

_____

_____

_____

Treatment:_____

_____

_____

_____

_____

_____

_____

_____

_____

_____

_____

_____

Medication/Dosage:_____

_____

_____

_____

_____

_____

Date_____   Dr:_____ Dr. Ph. No._____

Illness/Problem:_____
_____
_____
_____

Diagnosis:_____
_____
_____
_____
_____
_____
_____
_____
_____
_____
_____

Treatment:_____
_____
_____
_____
_____
_____
_____
_____
_____
_____
_____
_____
_____

Medication/Dosage:_____
_____
_____
_____
_____
_____

Date_____   Dr:_____ Dr. Ph. No._____

Illness/Problem:_____

_____

_____

_____

Diagnosis:_____

_____

_____

_____

_____

_____

_____

_____

_____

_____

Treatment:_____

_____

_____

_____

_____

_____

_____

_____

_____

_____

_____

_____

_____

Medication/Dosage:_____

_____

_____

_____

_____

_____

_____

Date_____   Dr:_____ Dr. Ph. No._____

Illness/Problem:_____
_____
_____
_____

Diagnosis:_____
_____
_____
_____
_____
_____
_____
_____
_____
_____

Treatment:_____
_____
_____
_____
_____
_____
_____
_____
_____
_____
_____
_____

Medication/Dosage:_____
_____
_____
_____
_____
_____

Date_____   Dr:_____ Dr. Ph. No._____

Illness/Problem:_____

_____

_____

_____

Diagnosis:_____

_____

_____

_____

_____

_____

_____

_____

Treatment:_____

_____

_____

_____

_____

_____

_____

_____

_____

_____

Medication/Dosage:_____

_____

_____

_____

_____

_____

Date_____   Dr:_____ Dr. Ph. No._____

Illness/Problem:_____
_____
_____
_____

Diagnosis:_____
_____
_____
_____
_____
_____
_____
_____
_____
_____

Treatment:_____
_____
_____
_____
_____
_____
_____
_____
_____
_____
_____
_____

Medication/Dosage:_____
_____
_____
_____
_____
_____

Date_____   Dr:_____ Dr. Ph. No._____

Illness/Problem:_____

_____

_____

_____

Diagnosis:_____

_____

_____

_____

_____

_____

_____

_____

_____

_____

Treatment:_____

_____

_____

_____

_____

_____

_____

_____

_____

_____

_____

_____

_____

Medication/Dosage:_____

_____

_____

_____

_____

_____

_____

Date_____   Dr:_____ Dr. Ph. No._____

Illness/Problem:_____

_____

_____

_____

Diagnosis:_____

_____

_____

_____

_____

_____

_____

_____

_____

_____

Treatment:_____

_____

_____

_____

_____

_____

_____

_____

_____

_____

_____

_____

Medication/Dosage:_____

_____

_____

_____

_____

_____

Date_____   Dr:_____ Dr. Ph. No._____

Illness/Problem:_____

_____

_____

_____

Diagnosis:_____

_____

_____

_____

_____

_____

_____

_____

_____

_____

Treatment:_____

_____

_____

_____

_____

_____

_____

_____

_____

_____

_____

_____

Medication/Dosage:_____

_____

_____

_____

_____

_____

Date_____   Dr:_____ Dr. Ph. No._____

Illness/Problem:_____
_____
_____
_____

Diagnosis:_____
_____
_____
_____
_____
_____
_____
_____
_____
_____

Treatment:_____
_____
_____
_____
_____
_____
_____
_____
_____
_____
_____
_____
_____

Medication/Dosage:_____
_____
_____
_____
_____
_____

Date_____   Dr:_____ Dr. Ph. No._____

Illness/Problem:_____

_____

_____

_____

Diagnosis:_____

_____

_____

_____

_____

_____

_____

_____

_____

Treatment:_____

_____

_____

_____

_____

_____

_____

_____

_____

_____

_____

Medication/Dosage:_____

_____

_____

_____

_____

_____

Date_____   Dr:_____ Dr. Ph. No._____

Illness/Problem:_____

_____

_____

_____

Diagnosis:_____

_____

_____

_____

_____

_____

_____

_____

_____

_____

_____

Treatment:_____

_____

_____

_____

_____

_____

_____

_____

_____

_____

_____

_____

_____

Medication/Dosage:_____

_____

_____

_____

_____

_____

_____

Date_____   Dr:_____ Dr. Ph. No._____

Illness/Problem:_____

_____

_____

_____

Diagnosis:_____

_____

_____

_____

_____

_____

_____

_____

_____

_____

_____

Treatment:_____

_____

_____

_____

_____

_____

_____

_____

_____

_____

_____

_____

_____

Medication/Dosage:_____

_____

_____

_____

_____

_____

Date_____   Dr:_____ Dr. Ph. No._____

Illness/Problem:_____
_____
_____
_____

Diagnosis:_____
_____
_____
_____
_____
_____
_____
_____
_____
_____

Treatment:_____
_____
_____
_____
_____
_____
_____
_____
_____
_____
_____
_____
_____

Medication/Dosage:_____
_____
_____
_____
_____
_____

Date_____   Dr:_____ Dr. Ph. No._____

Illness/Problem:_____
_____
_____
_____

Diagnosis:_____
_____
_____
_____
_____
_____
_____
_____
_____
_____

Treatment:_____
_____
_____
_____
_____
_____
_____
_____
_____
_____
_____
_____

Medication/Dosage:_____
_____
_____
_____
_____
_____

Date_____   Dr:_____ Dr. Ph. No._____

Illness/Problem:_____
_____
_____
_____

Diagnosis:_____
_____
_____
_____
_____
_____
_____
_____
_____
_____

Treatment:_____
_____
_____
_____
_____
_____
_____
_____
_____
_____
_____
_____

Medication/Dosage:_____
_____
_____
_____
_____
_____

Date_____   Dr:_____ Dr. Ph. No._____

Illness/Problem:_____

_____

_____

_____

Diagnosis:_____

_____

_____

_____

_____

_____

_____

_____

_____

Treatment:_____

_____

_____

_____

_____

_____

_____

_____

_____

_____

_____

Medication/Dosage:_____

_____

_____

_____

_____

_____

Date_____ Dr:_____ Dr. Ph. No._____

Illness/Problem:_____

_____

_____

_____

Diagnosis:_____

_____

_____

_____

_____

_____

_____

_____

_____

Treatment:_____

_____

_____

_____

_____

_____

_____

_____

_____

_____

_____

Medication/Dosage:_____

_____

_____

_____

_____

_____

Date_____   Dr:_____ Dr. Ph. No._____

Illness/Problem:_____
_____
_____
_____

Diagnosis:_____
_____
_____
_____
_____
_____
_____
_____
_____
_____
_____

Treatment:_____
_____
_____
_____
_____
_____
_____
_____
_____
_____
_____
_____
_____

Medication/Dosage:_____
_____
_____
_____
_____
_____
_____

Date_____   Dr:_____ Dr. Ph. No._____

Illness/Problem:_____
_____
_____
_____

Diagnosis:_____
_____
_____
_____
_____
_____
_____
_____
_____
_____
_____

Treatment:_____
_____
_____
_____
_____
_____
_____
_____
_____
_____
_____
_____
_____

Medication/Dosage:_____
_____
_____
_____
_____
_____

Date_____   Dr:_____ Dr. Ph. No._____

Illness/Problem:_____

_____

_____

_____

Diagnosis:_____

_____

_____

_____

_____

_____

_____

_____

_____

_____

Treatment:_____

_____

_____

_____

_____

_____

_____

_____

_____

_____

_____

_____

_____

Medication/Dosage:_____

_____

_____

_____

_____

_____

Date_____   Dr:_____ Dr. Ph. No._____

Illness/Problem:_____
_____
_____
_____

Diagnosis:_____
_____
_____
_____
_____
_____
_____
_____
_____
_____
_____

Treatment:_____
_____
_____
_____
_____
_____
_____
_____
_____
_____
_____
_____
_____

Medication/Dosage:_____
_____
_____
_____
_____
_____
_____

Date_____   Dr:_____ Dr. Ph. No._____

Illness/Problem:_____

_____

_____

_____

Diagnosis:_____

_____

_____

_____

_____

_____

_____

_____

_____

_____

Treatment:_____

_____

_____

_____

_____

_____

_____

_____

_____

_____

_____

_____

_____

Medication/Dosage:_____

_____

_____

_____

_____

_____

_____

List of Surgeries

Date	Surgery	Doctors	Reason	Possible Side Effects	Related Pages

Allergies – Date of First Occurrence

Date	Allergy/Allergic Reaction	Symptoms	Medication	Related Pages

Current Allergy	Date/Year First Occurrence	Medication/ Treatment	Related Pages

Family Health History

Date/Year(s)	Family Member	Maternal/Paternal/ Relationship	Illness	Outcome
-------	Ex: Anna Smith	Ex: Maternal Grandmother	Ex: Heart Problems	Ex: Heart Attack

List of Emergency Room Visits

Date/Time	Hospital	Ailment	Reason	Doctor(s)	Related Pages

List of Hospitalizations

Begin Date – End Date	Hospital	Ailment	Reason	Doctor(s)	Related Pages

Medical History Photos

(Paste photos along with dates/time.)

Medical History Photos

(Paste photos along with dates/time.)

Medical History Photos

(Paste photos along with dates/time.)

Medical History Photos

(Paste photos along with dates/time.)

Medical History Photos

(Paste photos along with dates/time.)

List of Natural Treatments

Date Acquired	Vitamins/Herbs/ Oils	Dosage	Reason for Taking	Additional Benefits	Current?

What would you like to see in future editions of this book?

Please e-mail me with future book update suggestions at: rugstudio@gmail.com . I would love to hear your ideas for new sections along with which sections you would like to see shorter or longer. Any ideas will be taken into consideration for future book updates!

Made in the USA
Middletown, DE
16 February 2016